Hyperbaric Oxygen Therapy

The Ultimate Beginner's Guide to Understanding the Hyperbaric Chamber

Table Of Contents

Introduction

This short book is for people who are interested in learning more about hyperbaric oxygen therapy and are not sure where to start or what information to rely on. I made this book in response to the high demand of people wanting to know more about hyperbaric oxygen therapy and why it has become so popular.

The Internet has many articles and a ton of misinformation regarding hyperbaric medicine that confuse people who are interested in learning about this revolutionary craze and want to possibly experience the effects for themselves. In this book, I am going to give you a short, concise guide for everything you need to know about hyperbaric chambers and help you decide if you should take the next step of trying one out.

This book contains proven steps and strategies on how to maximize the use of hyperbaric oxygen therapy (HBOT) in treating patients with different diseases and disorders, like decompression sickness, air embolism, gangrene and more. We will cover the history, benefits, contraindications, and everything else a beginner needs to know about hyperbaric medicine.

I recommend that you take notes while you are reading this book as it will ensure that you get the most out of the information in here. I want you to feel you have made a purchase that is worth your money and you can also look over the notes of this book even after you've finished reading it. The notes will help you to pinpoint exactly what you need to remember and by writing things down, you will be able to recall specifics during your sessions.

Lastly, remember that everything in this book has been compiled through research, my own experiences, as well as the experiences of others, so feel free to question what you have read in this book. I encourage you to do your own research on the things that you want to look deeper into. The more you understand about hyperbaric medicine and the chambers, the more educated your decision-making process will be when it comes to trying out a session or giving advice to others.

Chapter 1:

Overview of HBOT

In 2013, the World Health Organization (WHO) presented the five most common causes of mortality in the world; namely, Ischemic Heart Disease (12.6%), Cerebrovascular diseases (9.7%), Lower Respiratory Infections (6.8%), HIV/AIDS (4.9%), and Chronic Obstructive Pulmonary Disease (4.8%). Based on the statistics, cardiovascular diseases are the most prevalent, regardless of the age group or gender. Some of the cardiovascular disorders include angina pectoris, myocardial infarction, ischemia, heart failure, impaired vascular perfusion, and many more.

The prevalence of cardiovascular diseases is so high primarily because of sedentary lifestyle, unhealthy diet, stress, pollution, obesity, alcoholism, and smoking. Due to these diseases, the demand for healthcare has increased drastically over these past few years. As the trend continuously increases, various health aligned groups have been alarmed and have decided to come up with a campaign or advocacy to promote healthy lifestyles and clean living.

Herbal and dietary supplements have also been promoted in order to achieve the daily dietary requirements for the public. Various diets have been trending in an attempt to lose weight and fight obesity, such as the Atkins diet, Vegan diet, Mediterranean diet, and South Beach diet. Due to these advocacies, people have become more conscious in terms of their health and promoting longevity.

As people continuously seek ways to fight diseases, various treatment modalities have been discovered, invented, and introduced; this includes many types of alternative medicines. According to Merriam-Webster dictionary, alternative medicine is a system of healing or treating a disease in a way that is not included in the traditional medical curricula. This includes chiropractic, homeopathy, faith healing, herbal supplements, and others. Aside from these alternative medicines, various other therapies and treatment modalities have also been introduced to the public.

This increasing trend in health awareness has paved the way for the introduction of hyperbaric medicine, which is one of the most commonly used alternative treatment modalities. Hyperbaric medicine is also commonly known as the decompression chamber or recompression chamber, but most commonly referred to as hyperbaric oxygen therapy (HBO therapy). The word "hyperbaric" came from the Greek words, "hyper" meaning "over or above" and "baro" meaning "weight". Therefore, hyperbaric means above the weight, or simply, above the normal weight of the atmosphere.

HBO therapy is a procedure wherein one hundred percent of oxygen concentration is used and introduced into the lungs in order to hyper-oxygenate the blood for proper circulation and sufficient perfusion. In order to make the therapy effective, the procedure is performed at a level higher than the atmospheric pressure. Since most of the people are suffering from cardiovascular diseases, specifically perfusion problems, the demand for HBO therapy has increased.

In order to deliver one hundred percent oxygen, the procedure requires a pressure chamber as well as an oxygen source. During the procedure, the concentration of oxygen being administered is three times higher than the normal breathing oxygen at normal air pressure. Best of all, HBO therapy is proven to be safe, painless, affordable, and non-invasive.

Chapter 2:

History of Hyperbaric Medicine

The development of hyperbaric medicine started when Joseph Priestley, an English scientist, discovered oxygen in 1775. As soon as the oxygen was discovered, hyperbaric oxygen was introduced, but was prohibited due to a belief that it had some toxic effects on the Central Nervous System (CNS) and Respiratory System. Hyperbaric medicine had not been used until Orval J. Cunningham, Professor of Anesthesia at the University of Kansas, observed the correlation between altitude in the recovery of his patients to circulatory disorders. Most importantly, he discovered that his patients recovered faster when at sea level.

From this discovery, Cunningham started to consider the use of hyperbaric air in treating his patients. He started to test the effectiveness of hyperbaric air when he treated his patients who were suffering from the Spanish flu in 1918. Although the treatment was successful, it was disapproved by the American Medical Association because the evidence presented was believed to be insufficient and unacceptable.

Despite the disapproval from the AMA, Behnke and Shaw attempted to use hyperbaric medicine again to treat their patients with decompression sickness in 1937. The treatment was once again successful and it was the reason why Churchhill-Davidson also used hyperbaric oxygen to enhance the radio sensitivity of tumors in 1955.

Hyperbaric medicine became more popular when Ite Boerema used it in cardiac surgery in 1956. The idea of using HBO therapy in treating ischemic disorders began when Willem Hendrik Brummelkamp used it for treating gangrene in 1961.

Due to these significant findings, Henshaw, a British clergyman came up with the idea of creating a chamber that was capable of treating different diseases. This chamber was the first well-known chamber and was called "domocilum." Fontaine, a French surgeon, further improved hyperbaric medicine when he built and introduced a pressurized mobile operating room in 1879.

Needless to say, these findings and discoveries served as a spark to further ignite the flame of hyperbaric medicine. Despite these numerous discoveries, scientists are still curious about enhancing the technology of hyperbaric medicine in order to further benefit their patients.

Chapter 3:

The Science Behind HBOT

In order to understand how HBO therapy works for our bodies, we must first understand how the circulatory system works. HBO therapy works hand-in-hand with our body's circulatory system by helping the body circulate more oxygen to areas that need sufficient perfusion. This perfusion itself is the key to the treatment of a variety of cardiovascular problems.

Blood is mostly composed of red blood cells (RBC), white blood cells (WBC), hemoglobin, platelets, and plasma. Red blood cells are oxygen-carrying cells that are responsible for distributing oxygen throughout the body's tissues. White blood cells are responsible for fighting bacteria and viruses in order to prevent infection. Hemoglobin is the protein in red blood cells that carries oxygen, while blood clotting is the main role of platelets. Lastly, the component that constitutes almost half of the blood's volume is the plasma; the plasma holds the blood cells and is responsible for distributing them to all parts of the body.

Oxygen is needed by the body in order to promote tissue growth and healing. It allows aerobic metabolism that aids in the production of glucose, which is needed for energy. Without oxygen, cells would starve, tissues would degenerate, and the whole body's system would fail not long after.

Under normal conditions, when a person inhales oxygen either through his/her mouth or nose, it would go directly to the lungs where the gas exchange occurs. When the non-oxygenated blood reaches the lungs, specifically the alveoli, it will be replaced by oxygenated blood through the process of diffusion, and will circulate back through the body. Furthermore, the oxygen-rich blood will supply oxygen to the tissues and will circulate back to the lungs as non-oxygenated blood.

The purpose of HBO therapy is to increase the amount of oxygen that the tissues are receiving by increasing the amount of oxygen that the blood can carry. For conditions like anemia, the body is receiving insufficient oxygen because of decreased RBCs. HBO therapy will saturate the blood with oxygen in order to temporarily restore it to a normal level of blood gases, in order to promote sufficient tissue perfusion.

During an HBO session, 100 percent of oxygen is introduced into the lungs under an increased atmospheric pressure. Due to an increased pressure, the oxygen dissolves into plasma; thus, making it hyper-oxygenated. Since plasma covers most of the blood, the bloodstream is now capable of carrying more oxygen. With the help of an oxygen-rich RBC and hyper-oxygenated plasma, the tissue will now receive more oxygen as compared to normal blood circulation.

Since plasma is capable of seeping into different areas within the body, this would ensure that the tissues that are diminished and compromised will be well-perfused. Other than blood, plasma can also go into different body fluids, like cerebrospinal fluid (CSF), lymph nodes, and bone. HBO therapy also helps in fighting infection because it enhances the ability of WBC to kill bacteria.

Chapter 4:

Types of Hyperbaric Chambers

In order to deliver oxygen into the body, HBO therapy uses equipment called *chambers*. Hyperbaric chambers are made of high-quality materials to ensure correct oxygen administration. In order to ensure their quality, all hyperbaric chambers should have clearance from the Food and Drug Administration (FDA). The FDA conducts a thorough and careful quality check to ensure that the device is safe and effective.

There are four main types of chambers which are used depending on a person's condition, the advice of the physician, and the number of patients to be treated. Above all, the convenience of the patient is the primary criterion in deciding which chamber should be used. If the patient is claustrophobic, then he/she could consider the Multi-place Chambers. If the patient prefers to just lie down and relax, then he/she could use the Mono-place Chambers.

Four of the most common types of chambers are Smaller "Mono-place" Chambers, Multi-place Chambers, Duo-place Chambers, and Topical HBO therapy.

Smaller "Mono-place" Chamber

From the term itself, this chamber is "mono-place," meaning it can only accommodate one patient at a time. The chamber is about 7 feet long and requires the patient to be in a lying position. No medical staff is allowed to enter the chamber during the treatment. Mono-place chambers may be pressurized either with pure oxygen or compressed air. One of the most common effects of mono-place chambers are hyperoxic seizures, especially when the compressed air is used. A mask, or hood, is needed for compressed air administration, while pure oxygen no longer needs any equipment.

Since the patient is enclosed within the chamber and is left alone, this type of chamber may not be suited for patients with claustrophobia. Treatment for this disorder will be discussed later on. During the treatment, a trained technician must always stay and talk with the patient to avoid the patient getting afraid.

Multi-place Chamber

If two or more patients need to undergo the therapy simultaneously, then a multi-place chamber is the best option because it can accommodate up to 12 patients at a time. With the Multi-place chamber, a trained technician is now allowed to stay inside the unit to closely monitor the patient(s) and assist with the manipulation of equipment. In this chamber, the patient(s) may either lay down, sit, or walk. In order to receive the oxygen, a hood or mask may be worn, and can be pressurized to about 6 atmospheres of pressure.

Duo-place Chamber

This type of chamber can hold up to 2 people at a time and is quite similar to the mono-place chamber, just a little larger.

Topical HBOT

If the patient would like to focus on one specific part of the body, then he/she could consider the topical HBOT method. Topical HBOT involves application of gaseous oxygen to the affected part of the body (e.g. Wound, Gangrene). After the application, a plastic bag filled with 100 percent oxygen under pressure is wrapped around the area. This method is known to be the safest, easiest, fastest, and most affordable one.

Chapter 5:

Preparing for Therapy

Indications

HBOT was initially used for divers who suffered from decompression sickness, but as scientists continued to explore the advantages of hyperbaric medicine, new diseases are being treated and a wider variety of patients are benefitting. If you think you may have one of these conditions, then you should consult with your doctor because you could be a perfect candidate for HBO therapy.

Here are the key indications for HBO therapy:

<u>Air or Gas Embolism</u>

This is a condition in which large air bubbles get clogged within the blood vessels, causing impaired blood perfusion. HBO therapy decreases the size of the emboli and helps pull it out of the bloodstream before it causes any more damage.

<u>Carbon Monoxide Poisoning</u>

Hemoglobin has high affinity to carbon monoxide, which completely replaces oxygen. The therapy helps oxygen bind with hemoglobin again and aids in circulating the oxygen, while hemoglobin is still incapable.

<u>Exceptional blood loss (Anemia)</u>

HBO therapy helps people to overcome anemia by normalizing the levels of blood gases to allow sufficient oxygen perfusion.

Intracranial Abscess

HBO therapy ensures that intracranial tissues are still receiving sufficient oxygen. It also gives WBC the ability to fight the abscess.

Cyanide Poisoning

This condition is related to carbon monoxide poisoning and HBO therapy works to create the same effect in both.

Soft tissue and bony necrosis caused by delayed radiation

Necrosis is caused by hypoxic tissues. HBO therapy supplies oxygen to the necrotic tissues; thus, allowing regeneration.

Idiopathic Sudden Deafness

HBO therapy ensures sufficient blood circulation in the ear and can help combat idiopathic sudden deafness.

Venous, Arterial, and Pressure Ulcers

HBO therapy keeps the affected area well-oxygenated in order to promote wound healing and to prevent necrosis (as mentioned earlier).

Decompression Sickness

A condition most commonly experienced by divers, the exchange of their blood gases often become impaired. HBO therapy helps to normalize the blood gas exchange throughout the body.

<u>Others Include:</u>

Traumatic brain injuries

Clostridal Myositis and Myonecrosis (Gas Gangrene)

Diabetic Foot, Retinopathy, and/or Nephropathy

Necrotizing soft tissue infections

Certain types of burns

Certain types of brain or sinus infections

Although all forms of HBO therapy are safe and non-invasive, it is still important to check if you are fit for this type of treatment in order to prevent possible adverse effects. Moreover, HBO therapy is not a permanent replacement for your vitamins and regular medicines; most of the time, physicians recommend that you do HBO therapy together with your medicines.

Contraindications

Since hyperbaric oxygen therapy requires a pressure higher than the normal atmospheric pressure, this creates tension in the tissues that may be contraindicated with some medical conditions. If you are anxious of the possible complications, then you will have to consult your physician right away so that he/she can give you recommendations.

There have been reports that HBO therapy can cause exacerbation or relapse of some medical conditions and that is why the hyperbaric specialists should be very careful in assessing the patient. He/she should consider all the possible factors that could further compromise the patient's condition(s).

Untreated Pneumothorax and Chronic Obstructive Pulmonary Disease (COPD) are the absolute contraindications to HBOT. Pneumothorax is a condition in which the lungs are over-filled with air, causing tension in the lung cavity, while COPD is the obstruction of air pathways, either by mucus or constricted bronchioles.

In some cases, these two conditions could lead to tension pneumothorax due to a sudden increase in pressure within the lungs. Patients with asthma are also not allowed to undergo the hyperbaric oxygen therapy because it could progress into tension pneumothorax.

As mentioned earlier, there have been reports that patients with claustrophobia had a hard time staying inside the chamber. Physicians may advise taking benzodiazepines to tranquilize the patient during the treatment. If seizure is expected or if the patient has a history of seizures, then benzodiazepines could also be administered. Again, proper medical precautions should be observed during this process.

Furthermore, the patient should also inform his/her physician about the medicines they are taking because they may also be contraindicated with the therapy. The physician may either ask the patient to discontinue the therapy or require him/her to discontinue the medicines a few days prior to the treatment.

If you are taking one of these medicines, then you can not be treated with HBO therapy:

Doxorubicin (Adriamycin)

Cisplatin

Disulfiram (Antabuse)

Mafenide Acetate (Sulfamylon)

Bleomycin

Doxorubicin

Other than the contraindications, there are also *relative contraindications,* which means that the therapy could still be continued, but with special considerations. The following medical conditions are *relative contraindications*:

COPD with Air Trapping

Cardiac diseases

Patients with a history of chest surgery

Malignant Diseases (example: Cancer)

Hyperpyrexia (High fever)

Upper Respiratory infections

Emphysema with Carbon Dioxide retention

Middle Ear Barotrauma

Eustachian Tube Dysfunction

Pacemakers or Epidural Pain Pump

Studies show that HBO therapy has no relative side effects for pregnant patients. Fetal hemoglobin has high affinity to carbon monoxide, which lowers the threshold in pregnant patients for HBO therapy; thus, minimizing the risk of toxicity. Although there are no reported side effects, physicians should still be cautious about the dose and duration of the treatment to ensure safety for both the mother and the fetus.

Preparation

Since HBOT uses pure oxygen, it is highly flammable, which is why it is important to make sure that you don't carry any items that could ignite a fire, such as lighters, battery powered devices, and hair and wound-care products that are potentially flammable. The patient is only allowed to wear clean cotton clothing in the chamber to prevent friction. Dentures, jewelry, and other personal garments should be taken off before entering the chamber. Oil or alcohol-based grooming products, such as hairspray, makeup, and perfume should also be taken off.

All medications that are contraindicated with the treatment should be discontinued a few days before the treatment, or depending on the order of the physician. In order to ensure correct evaluation by the physician, you should provide a complete list of all the medications you have taken three months prior to the treatment. Patients are also advised to stop consuming alcohol and carbonated drinks four hours prior to treatment; they may also be advised to stop smoking on the course of treatment to prevent interfering with the proper oxygen circulation.

The patient should also be educated on what he/she will feel like during the treatment in order to prevent fear and anxiety. Typically the patient will feel a sensation similar to that felt while flying or landing in an airplane. They should also be advised that the pressure that will be felt in the ears is normal, and as soon as the pressure is released, the ears will automatically "pop".

Needless to say, certain diagnostic tests may be required to determine if hyperbaric therapy is right for you. One of the most common tests is the transcutaneous oxygen measurement in order to determine the oxygen levels in your body. Also, all patients are required to undergo a Chest X-Ray to rule out pneumothorax or other such respiratory diseases.

It is also important to maintain an open communication with your physician in order to freely express fear and anxiety. The physician should address all the questions that the patient has before treatment; he/she must also make sure that the patient fully understands what the procedure is, what will happen during the procedure, and what he/she should do before, during, and after the procedure.

Cost

Hyperbaric medicine is more affordable than many other treatment modalities and that is one of the reasons why many patients prefer this type of treatment. HBO therapy can be done either as an out-patient or in-patient treatment. The cost depends on the duration and the type of chamber the patient will be using. However, for a rough estimate, HBO therapy typically costs around $108 to $250 for a one-hour treatment in private clinics, and can cost up to $1,000 (on the high end) when done in some hospitals.

Chapter 6:

During the Treatment

The treatment is generally painless and non-invasive, although the patient may feel some discomfort during the treatment due to an increase in pressure. To ensure the patient's comfort, the physician may allow the patient to read, sleep, listen to music, or rest comfortably while inside the chamber. An air conditioner is also equipped because the changes in pressure also change the temperature inside the chamber which could be another cause of possible discomfort. The patient is asked to take periodic deep breaths to remain calm.

The treatment has two phases: The pressurization and the decompression. During pressurization, the oxygen is being delivered into the patient's lungs at an increased pressure. The pressure used varies from 2.4 Atmospheres Absolute Pressure (ATA) up to 6 ATA. The pressure is then released through a valve during decompression. At this point, the changes in pressure due to these phases may cause discomfort in the ears. The patient may feel pressure in his/her ears during pressurization, but will immediately "squeak" or "pop" during decompression.

The discomfort in the ear is relieved by doing the Valsalva maneuver or "jaw wiggling". According to the Merriam-Webster dictionary, Valsalva maneuver is a forceful attempt at expiration while holding the nostrils closed and keeping the mouth shut. The maneuver relieves the discomfort in the ears by releasing the pressure.

Since pressurization causes an increase in temperature, it is important to monitor the patient's body temperature to prevent hyperthermia. Consequently, the patient should be kept warm by doing a tepid sponge bath during decompression to prevent hypothermia.

Luckily, the rate of pressurization and decompression can be adjusted based on the condition and tolerance of the patient. The therapy may last for one to eight hours, during which, the health care team continuously monitors the patient for any possible adverse reaction to his/her body. For wound healing, the treatment may last for two hours; for acute conditions like carbon monoxide poisoning, it may last for four hours; and for diving injuries, it may last up to eight hours.

HBOT with a Mono-place chamber

The administration of oxygen is easier with a Mono-place chamber because it is already pressurized. The chamber has a padded table that slides into a clear plastic tube, in which the patient lies down in a reclining position. To prevent fear or claustrophobia, the chamber is made with clear acrylic that allows the patient to look at the outside, and allows the trained technician to closely monitor the patient. While in the chamber, a gentle "hiss" will be heard as soon as the oxygen comes through the chamber.

HBOT with a Multi-place Chamber

As mentioned earlier in this book, Multi-place chambers come with hoods and helmets to ensure sufficient administration of oxygen. Patients breath 100 percent oxygen to maximize the treatment, but may have "air breaks" to breath in room air at 21 percent oxygen in order to prevent oxygen toxicity. Unlike Mono-place chambers, patients are allowed to lie down, sit, or walk inside of Multi-place chambers.

Chapter 7:

After the Treatment

Complications

Just like most treatments, HBOT comes with some risk. The treatment may cause trauma and exhaustion in the body of the patient because of the increase and fluctuation of pressure. The changes in pressure could "squeeze" the tissues, causing the air to be trapped inside the body's cavities, such as the dental fillings, paranasal sinuses, eardrums, and the lungs. The trapped air could cause tension in the tissues, which induce conditions such as middle and inner ear injuries, eardrum rupture, and leakage of fluid.

The increase in pressure may also cause damage to some organs. In the eyes, cataracts may develop due to an increased optic pressure. In the cardiovascular system, HBO therapy may exacerbate congestive heart failure. Congestive Heart Failure is a condition in which the heart gets too congested with blood either because of impaired contraction or valve problems. The pressure from HBO therapy may further congest the heart so much that it could lead to heart failure.

Since HBO therapy also hyperoxygenates the blood, it could also cause oxygen toxicity, which is characterized by blurring of vision, swelling of the lens, tinnitus (ringing in the ears), facial twitches, nausea, dizziness, and irritability. The central nervous system (CNS) could also be affected by oxygen toxicity, which is characterized by seizures and light-headedness. The toxicity could also cause either blindness secondary to Optic Neuritis (Optic Nerve Inflammation) or myopia (nearsightedness).

Oxygen toxicity may also affect the respiratory system. Symptoms are dry cough, chest pain or burning, and decreased vital capacity. Although the complications may sound alarming, most of them are temporary and may resolve after a few minutes.

Other than the aforementioned complications, here are the other complications that need urgent intervention by physicians:

Eustachian Tube Dysfunction – Characterized by ear pain, fullness, and muffled hearing

Sinus pain or bleeding

Tooth pain

Nystagmus

Vertigo

Diet

There are no specific dietary requirements for patients who undergo hyperbaric oxygen therapy. However, the patients are encouraged to eat high-fiber foods in order to prevent straining that could further increase the pressure within the body. It is also commonly advised to eat foods that are rich in Vitamin C, in order to aid in tissue regeneration and wound healing.

Food rich in Iron is also encouraged in order to maintain normal blood levels. The patient should eat fruits and vegetables in order to meet vitamin and mineral requirements. As you might have expected, the recovery of the patient from his/her condition will be faster if the hyperbaric oxygen therapy is supplemented with a healthy diet.

Duration

Depending on the condition, diagnosis, and the body response of the patient, the physician may require more than one session for the therapy to become effective. For carbon monoxide poisoning, the patient may be asked to go for three visits, while non-healing wounds can require up to 25 to 30 treatments. The patient may receive one treatment per day, usually every weekday, for 20 to 30 days.

Chapter 8:

Advancements in Hyperbaric Medicine

From the simple decompression sickness to the treatment of gangrene, necrotic tissues, and ischemic diseases, it is no wonder why hyperbaric medicine developed throughout the years. As scientists continue to explore the other benefits of the treatment, there is no doubt that in future years, HBO therapy will cover newer medical conditions. Advancements in hyperbaric medicine does not only focus on the diseases, it also focuses on improving the quality of the chambers in order to provide the best experience possible.

The hard-shelled pressure vessel is the most traditional type of hyperbaric chamber. This chamber can be run at absolute pressures as much as 87 PSI or 600,000 Pa. A recent advancement in the hyperbaric chamber industry is the manufacturing of portable or "soft" chambers that operate between 4.4 and 7.3 PSI.

There are also certain conditions that are not yet proven to be responsive with the hyperbaric oxygen therapy. Some of these are Autism, Cancer, Diabetes, Human Immunodeficiency Virus (HIV) or Acquired Immunodeficiency Syndrome, Asthma, Bell's and Cerebral Palsy, Multiple Sclerosis, Migraines, Depression, Heart disease, Parkinson's diseases, spinal cord injuries, and stroke. Other diseases include Allergies, Arthritis, Chronic Fatigue Syndrome, Fibromyalgia, Gastrointestinal Ulcers and Cirrhosis.

Needless to say, it is an exciting time because scientists are working to see if they can find the cures to these serious diseases through HBOT. We will just have to wait and see.

Conclusion

I hope this book was able to help you learn more about hyperbaric medicine, what it is useful for, the different options you have, and the positive and negative effects of using a hyperbaric chamber. Now that you have learned the important factors regarding hyperbaric medicine, you can finally decide if you want to try a session with the help of a professional.

Plus, a little addition to your knowledge base does not hurt. It's good to know about new innovations because it keeps you in the know and up-to-date in a world where every big city has hyperbaric chambers popping up for public use.

Finally, if you enjoyed this book, please take the time to share your thoughts and send me a message or even post a review to Amazon.

Thank you and good luck!

Made in the USA
Las Vegas, NV
07 March 2022